Anne TOGO
Bakary DIARRA
Akory AG IKNANE

Antibiotic prescribing in pediatrics

Anne TOGO
Bakary DIARRA
Akory AG IKNANE

Antibiotic prescribing in pediatrics

In children under 5

ScienciaScripts

Imprint

Any brand names and product names mentioned in this book are subject to trademark, brand or patent protection and are trademarks or registered trademarks of their respective holders. The use of brand names, product names, common names, trade names, product descriptions etc. even without a particular marking in this work is in no way to be construed to mean that such names may be regarded as unrestricted in respect of trademark and brand protection legislation and could thus be used by anyone.

Cover image: www.ingimage.com

This book is a translation from the original published under ISBN 978-620-6-71237-4.

Publisher:
Sciencia Scripts
is a trademark of
Dodo Books Indian Ocean Ltd. and OmniScriptum S.R.L publishing group

120 High Road, East Finchley, London, N2 9ED, United Kingdom
Str. Armeneasca 28/1, office 1, Chisinau MD-2012, Republic of Moldova, Europe
Printed at: see last page
ISBN: 978-620-7-65581-6

ANNE TOGO, BAKARY DIARRA, AKORY AG IKNANE

PRESCRIPTION OF ANTIBIOTICS IN PAEDIATRICS IN THE DISTRICT OF BAMAKO

AUTHORS

ANNE TOGO, General Pharmacist, Faculty of Pharmacy at the University of Science, Techniques and Technologies in Bamako, having completed her doctoral thesis in the field of nutrition under the supervision of Professor Akory AG IKNANE and Dr Bakary Diarra. She has completed internships at the National Health Laboratory (LNS), the Mali Hospital laboratory and several pharmacies.

BAKARY DIARRA, public health physician, qualitative scientist, assistant professor of public health at the Faculty of Medicine and Odontostomatology in Bamako. He is currently Head of the Nutrition and Food Safety Department at the Institut National de Santé Publique (INSP), and has been Secretary General of Health, Director General of the Agence Nationale d'Évaluation des Hôpitaux (ANEH), and District and Community Health Centre Chief Medical Officer?

Akory AG IKNANE, Professor of Public Health and Nutrition, Head of the Nutrition Masters at the Faculty of Medicine and Odontostomatology in Bamako, WHO consultant for health emergencies, health system strengthening, training, research and innovation, Chairman of the Malian Nutrition Network (REMANUT), Secretary General of the Société Malienne de Santé Publique (SOMASAP) and Editor-in-Chief of the scientific journal, Mali Santé Publique, former Director General of the Institut National de Santé Publique (INSP), the Agence Nationale pour la Sécurité Sanitaire des Aliments (ANSSA) and the Agence Nationale d'Investissement des collectivités Territoriales du Mali (ANICT) - Bamako (Mali).

BACKGROUND AND JUSTIFICATION

Antibiotics are medicines used to treat bacterial infections. They can kill bacteria or prevent them from reproducing, allowing the body's natural defences to eliminate them (1).

The era of antibiotics began in earnest in 1941, following the industrial production of penicillins discovered in 1929 by Flemming (2). A large number of existing ATBs are made up of natural molecules, manufactured by micro-organisms: fungi or other bacteria (3). But the ease with which they can be used, and the habit of treating infectious diseases with them, have led to the routine use of antibiotics in clinical circumstances which, more often than not, do not justify them (4).

Maintaining the effectiveness of antibiotics for the treatment of infectious diseases is essential for achieving some or all of the sustainable development goals. At the same time, it is important to achieve the goals of reducing antibiotic resistance (5).

In sub-Saharan Africa, the mortality rate linked to antimicrobial resistance is estimated at 27.3 deaths per year per 100,000 inhabitants(6). A study conducted in the paediatrics department of Burkina Faso's national hospital centre showed a 79.1% rate of antibiotic prescriptions in children under one year of age (7).

Antibiotic treatments have increased life expectancy by more than ten years, more than any other medical treatment. However, the widespread, even abusive, use of certain antibiotics, including as preventive or curative treatments or as food supplements in animal feed, in fish farming, in veterinary and human medicine, or even as pesticides for treating plants (against fire blight, for example) has introduced a selection pressure that has led to the development of populations of antibiotic-resistant micro-organisms and a general decline in therapeutic efficacy (3).

Faced with the scale of the problem, the World Health Organization (WHO), at its World Assembly held in May 2015, adopted a Global Action Plan (GAP) to combat antimicrobial resistance, which sets out five objectives. This Action Plan emphasises the need for an effective "one world, one health" approach, involving coordination across many sectors and international actors, including human and veterinary medicine, agriculture, finance, the environment and well-informed consumers. The WHO then invited member countries to implement the measures proposed in the Global Action Plan to Combat Antimicrobial Resistance, adapting them to national priorities and specific circumstances to draw up a National Action Plan (NAP). Objective 4 of this plan is to optimise the use of antimicrobial medicines in human and animal health (8), and objective 5 is to make sustainable investments to combat antimicrobial resistance (9).

The widespread introduction of antibiotics after the Second World War was one of the most important therapeutic advances of the twentieth century. In hospitals, this has led to an increase in nosocomial risk, due to the lack of appropriate treatment for certain particularly resistant germs (10).

As well as increasing resistance, antibiotics can have well-described side-effects for individual patients: early exposure to antibiotics is associated with short-term effects such as an increased risk of invasive candidiasis, necrotising enterocolitis, late-onset sepsis and death, but also with allergic disease, obesity, diabetes and inflammatory bowel disease later in life, probably due to changes in the infant microbiome (11). In paediatric emergency departments, infectious pathology is a frequent reason for admission, and antibiotics are therefore frequently prescribed, most often for acute respiratory infections.

These prescriptions are not without clinical and epidemiological consequences, because even though they are well-tolerated, they are likely to cause undesirable side-effects on an individual level, and collectively, they contribute to the selection pressure leading to an increase in bacterial resistance to the most commonly used referents (12) . As a result, these micro-organisms are adapting to antibiotics, whose efficacy against infections for which they were previously active has diminished considerably. This phenomenon, known as bacterial resistance to antibiotics, is a real public health problem today, associated with a significant socio-economic burden (13). Over-consumption and misuse of antibiotics, as well as sub-optimal infection prevention practices, are responsible for the development of antibiotic resistance. Global consumption of antibiotics increased by 65% between 2000 and 2015, fuelled by a surge in use in middle- and low-income countries, which represents a threat to global health.Antibiotic resistance, caused by the consumption of antibiotics, is a growing threat to health. Global antibiotic consumption in 2015 was estimated at 42.3 billion defined daily doses(14). The health consequences and economic costs of antimicrobial resistance (AMR) are estimated at 10 million human deaths per year and a 2 to 3.5% drop in global gross domestic product (GDP), or USD 100,000 billion by 2050 (15).Today, this resistance is one of the most serious threats to global health, food security and development. It can affect anyone, at any age and in any country (9), so the rational use of antibiotics prescribed empirically or probabilistically in the absence of laboratory evidence is one of the essential measures for preventing the emergence of multi-resistant germs. Several causes have been described as being responsible for the emergence of bacterial resistance to antibiotics. These include the inappropriate and indiscriminate use of antibiotics. These bacteria, by becoming insensitive to any treatment, limit the range of antibiotics available in medical therapeutics. The situation is all the more alarming in that infections caused by resistant bacteria often lead to a prolongation of the pathological state and an increase in the mortality rate. The acquisition of these multiple resistances has led to a loss of efficacy in antibiotic therapy, ultimately leading to a therapeutic impasse (13).

However, their use requires a great deal of rigour, as incorrect handling can increase their disadvantages, in particular the occurrence of side-effects, the risk of unnecessary expenditure, and above all the spread of bacterial resistance. In hospitals, the disadvantages of antibiotic therapy are compounded by a higher rate of prescribing, more serious pathologies and a higher incidence of multi-resistant germs (7).

In Mali, as in many other developing countries, antibiotics are frequently prescribed on a probabilistic and uncontrolled basis, due to the shortage of biological analysis laboratories, whose services are beyond the means of local households, and therefore affect the early performance of specific microbiological tests; there is also the unavailability and financial inaccessibility of certain antibiotics selected for antibiotic susceptibility testing, if carried out. All this has a definite impact on the quality of medical prescribing in general, and antibiotic prescribing in particular. This is compounded by longer hospital stays(16). This bacterial resistance to antibiotics poses the problem of the choice of antibiotic therapy (17).

Since their discovery, antibiotics have provided invaluable services in infectious pathology. Certain infections caused by sensitive germs have become very rare, even if they have not completely disappeared. Knowledge of the rules for prescribing antibiotics helps to limit inappropriate prescribing, but it is essential to take stock of the situation before taking any therapeutic measures. With this in mind, we asked ourselves the following questions: (i) Does the prescribing of antibiotics to children under 5 years of age in paediatric wards in the District of Bamako comply with the National Standards? and (ii) What factors influence the quality of this prescribing of antibiotics? It was in response to these questions that the present study of antibiotic prescribing in children under 5 years of age in paediatric wards in the district of Bamako was initiated. In response to this problem, we will make a general assessment of the quality of antibiotic prescribing for children under 5 years of age in paediatric wards in the district of Bamako, based on a description of the socio-professional characteristics of prescribers, and a typology of prescriptions in paediatric wards, in order to determine compliance, identify factors influencing the quality of this prescribing and guide prescribing options for children.

GENERAL INFORMATION ON PATHOGENS AND ANTIBIOTICS

General information on bacteria

A bacterium is a single-celled organism with a very simple structure, no nucleus or organelles, diffuse genetic material, generally no chlorophyll, and reproduces by scissiparity. Bacteria generally measure between 0.1 and 50 micrometres. They can be curved or elongated, spherical or spiral (18).

Characteristics of the structure of bacteria (19).

The **walls of** bacteria are made up of a rigid envelope which ensures the integrity of the bacteria and is therefore responsible for the shape of the cells. It protects against variations in osmotic pressure. The part common to all bacterial walls is peptidoglycan (or murein), the innermost envelope. The composition of the wall varies according to species and bacterial group.

In Gram+ bacteria, the cell wall consists mainly of peptidoglycan. It contains teichoic acid (T.A.) bound to peptidoglycan and membrane lipids. Lipoteichoic acids (LT) retain the violet in the Gram stain.
The Gram- cell wall is much more complex. The peptidoglycan is thin and not very dense. The essential constituent is lipid A coupled to glucosamine and phosphorus residues. Phospholipids and embedded proteins are present, ensuring cohesion with the membrane, binding with peptidoglycan and permeability or non-permeability. Porins are essential to the life of bacteria, but also to the action of ATBs.

The plasma membrane is an internal structure at the interface between the cytoplasm and external structures. It has a trilamellar structure consisting of a phospholipid bilayer associated with proteins. The main functions of the plasma membrane are selective permeability and transport, respiration and excretion of hydrolytic enzymes.

The cytoplasm contains soluble RNA (messenger RNA and transfer RNA) and ribosomes, around 15,000 ribosomes made up of ribosomal proteins and RNA divided into subunits. A wide variety of inclusions exist in the cytoplasm. They serve to store organic or inorganic reserves.

The nuclear apparatus consists of the chromosome of the prokaryotic cell, located in an irregularly shaped region called the nucleoid. The chromosome is usually unique. It is the carrier of genetic information. It is a circular (sometimes linear) double helix, supercoiled by topoisomerases. It is made up of DNA (60%), RNA (30%) and proteins (10%). Extra-chromosomal DNA is not essential for life.

Plasmids are double-stranded DNA molecules that replicate independently of the chromosome, can be integrated into it and are transmissible. They carry fertility traits (F factor) and antibiotic resistance traits (R factor).

Transposable elements are fragments of DNA that move within the bacterial genome by transposition, hence the name transposon. The transposon is incapable of replication. Bacterial ribosomes comprise two subunits, 50S and 30S. Functionally, there are two sites for protein synthesis. The Aminoacyl site hosts the acyl-tRNA and the peptidyl site hosts the amino acid chain that is being formed. Some antibiotics interfere with protein synthesis at these two sites.

Some bacteria have inconstant structures. This is the inconsistent capsule, superficial, made up of acid polysaccharides. It is linked to certain pathogenic powers, as it prevents phagocytosis. It can be found in a soluble state in body fluids. It is involved in infraspecific identification. This typing is one of the methods used to recognise epidemics.

Glycocalyxes are extremely common polysaccharide polymers that surround bacteria and are difficult to visualise, except by electron microscopy. Glycocalyx is also called slime because it engulfs cells. It is responsible for the attachment of bacteria to cells and inert supports.

Flagella are proteins. They are anchored in the cytoplasm by a complex structure. They play a role in mobility and in the antigenic power used to differentiate bacterial species.

Pili or fimbriae are rigid, fibrillar structures located on the surface of Gram-bacteria and, exceptionally, Gram+ bacteria. These structures are finer than flagella. There are two types: common pili, which can specifically attach bacteria to the surface of eukaryotic cells, and sexual pili encoded by plasmids (factor F), which play a role in the attachment of bacteria to each other and in bacterial adhesion.

The bacterial spore is the survival form of the bacterium. It is present in a vegetative form that is metabolically active and potentially pathogenic or metabolically inactive and non-pathogenic (spore form). The transformation of the vegetative form into a spore is known as sporulation.

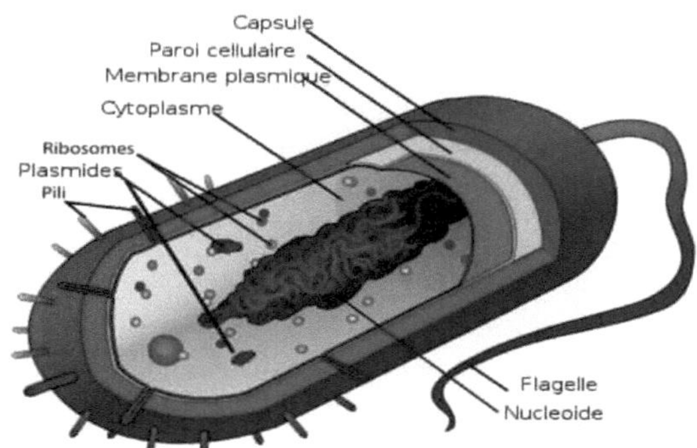

Figure 1: Structure of a bacterium (20).

General information on antibiotics

Antibiotics are chemical substances, natural or synthetic, which have a specific action on micro-organisms: bacteria or protozoa. When these molecules are capable of killing them, they are said to be **bactericidal**, and when they are limited to preventing their proliferation, they are said to be **bacteriostatic** (21).

Historically, the first antibiotic to be identified was penicillin. Although Ernest Duchesne had already discovered the curative properties of Penicillium glaucum at the end of the 19th century [e], the discovery of penicillin can be attributed to Sir Alexander Fleming, who realised in 1928 that some of his bacterial cultures in forgotten dishes had been contaminated by the experiments of his benchmate studying the fungus Penicillium notatum, and that the latter was inhibiting their reproduction. But the importance of this discovery, its implications and its medical uses were only understood and developed after its rediscovery, between the two world wars, particularly following the work of Howard Walter Florey, Ernst Chain and Norman Heatley in 1939.
In 1932, Gerhard Domagk at Bayer AG developed Prontosil, a sulphonamide, the first synthetic antibiotic. However, it was the subsequent discovery at the Institut Pasteur, in the therapeutic chemistry laboratory run by Ernest Fourneau, of the antibiotic properties of sulphanilamide, the active agent in Prontosil, (a discovery published in 1935 by Jacques and Thérèse Tréfouel, Federico Nitti and Daniel Bovet) that effectively paved the way for sulphamidotherapy. This

first synthetic antibiotic opened up a new way of combating many diseases that had previously been considered incurable.(22) . In 1939, René Dubos isolated tyrothricin (a mixture of tyrocidin and gramicidin) from Bacillus brevis, whose antibacterial action he had observed. Although gramicidin was indeed the first antibiotic to be marketed, its use was limited to topical application; toxic when administered intravenously, gramicidin proved highly effective during the Second World War in healing wounds and ulcers. As Howard Florey himself later recalled, the discovery of gramicidin was a decisive step in that it encouraged research into the therapeutic applications of penicillin, which had suffered several setbacks up until then. In 1944, Selman A. Waksman, Albert Schatz and E. Bugie discovered streptomycin, the first antibiotic to have an effect on Koch's bacillus, making it possible to treat tuberculosis. In 1952, erythromycin, the first known macrolide, newly isolated by J.M. McGuire of Eli Lilly, was marketed under the brand name Ilosone. Vancomycin was discovered in 1956. This was followed by the development of quinolones from 1962 onwards, and their derivatives, the fluoroquinolones, in the 1980s.At the beginning of the 1970s, research into antibiotics slowed sharply, as the therapeutic arsenal of the time made it possible to treat most bacterial infections effectively. In 2000, linezolid (approved by the FDA on 18 April 2000) was placed on the American market due to the emergence of resistance. Linezolid belongs to a new class of compounds known as oxazolidinones (3).

Classification of antibiotics

Antibiotics can be classified according to their origin, structure, mechanism and spectrum of activity.

Classification according to origin

There are three main groups of antibiotics:

- Natural antibiotics, produced by micro-organisms: Lower fungi such as Penicillium and Cephalosporium; Bacillus bacteria and especially Streptomyces (90% of antibiotics are produced by Streptomyces);
- Hemi-synthetic or semi-synthetic antibiotics: they result from the chemical transformation of natural compounds;
- Artificial antibiotics: obtained by chemical synthesis (22).

Classification by structure (23)

Molecules with the same basic chemical structure can be found in the same family, although some of them often have only one or two members: the following families can be distinguished

1. Beta-lactams (β-lactams) or β-lactam antibiotics

The beta-lactams are a family of antibiotics which are structurally very similar, as they all contain a **beta-lactam** core:

Penicillins

Penicillins are classified into 5 main categories

Penicillin G (benzylpenicillin) is a natural penicillin that is sensitive to penicillinases and is administered parenterally. They are the antibiotics of choice for ENT infections (strep throat), bronchial infections and soft tissue infections (boils, carbuncles, gangrene). Benzylpenicillin is still used in combination for septicaemia, endocarditis and meningitis. It is also used to treat syphilis and certain localised or generalised infections caused by sensitive germs.

Penicillins V (phenoxymethylpenicillin) are natural penicillins that are sensitive to penicillinases. They are still indicated for streptococcal infections (erysipelas, scarlet fever, etc.) and pneumococcal infections.

Penicillin M (oxacillin, cloxacillin). These penicillins are resistant to penicillinases due to their chemical structure, which gives them steric hindrance. They are used to treat infections caused by sensitive staphylococci, whether localised (ENT, pulmonary, bone) or generalised, and infections caused by staphylococci and/or streptococcus A. Oxacillin-based specialities were withdrawn from the market in May 2011 due to their unfavourable benefit-risk ratio.

Penicillin A or aminopenicillins (amoxicillin, ampicillin). They are widely used to treat localised infections (ENT, lung, etc.) or generalised infections, as well as to treat a wide range of diseases. than many other infections. Their combination with aminoglycosides is justified in severe infections.

Ureidopenicillins are effective against gram-negative germs

Carbapenems (Imipenem, Meropenem, Ertapenem, Doripenem). These injectable antibiotics are reserved for severe infections.

Monobactams (Aztreonam): This antibiotic is indicated for a range of adult infections: genitourinary, bronchopulmonary, septicaemic, cutaneous, intra-abdominal and gynaeco-obstetric.

2. Cephalosporins

Cephalosporins are antibiotics closely related to penicillins. They have a similar mechanism of action, but share the structure of 7-aminocephalosporanic acid. They are divided into three groups: 1st, 2nd and 3rd generation.

1st generation cephalosporins (C1G): cefaclor, cefadroxil, cefalexin, cefatrizine, cefazolin and cefradine. They are indicated for acute or recurrent ENT, respiratory and urinary tract infections caused by sensitive germs.

2nd generation cephalosporins (C2G): cefuroxime and cefoxitin are characterised by resistance to hydrolysis by beta-lactamases. These drugs should only be prescribed on the basis of an antibiogram for C1G-resistant infections.

3rd generation cephalosporins (C3G): Cefotaxime, Cefpodoxime, Ceftriaxone, Cefixime, Ceftazidime, Cefotiam, Cefepime, Cefpirome are indicated for the treatment of infections resistant to other beta-lactam antibiotics. Cephalosporins may be used in pregnant or breast-feeding women with limited adverse effects.

3. Beta-lactamase inhibitors

Amoxicillin is sometimes combined with clavulanic acid to prevent its destruction by certain bacteria. Example: Amoxicillin + clavulanic acid, Ticarcillin + clavulanic acid. Beta-lactamase inhibitors are suicide substrates that bind irreversibly to the beta-lactamase, thereby preserving the activity of the beta-lactam associated with it. Mainly gastrointestinal side effects, such as diarrhoea. Taking it with a meal and combining it with probiotics would limit this undesirable effect.

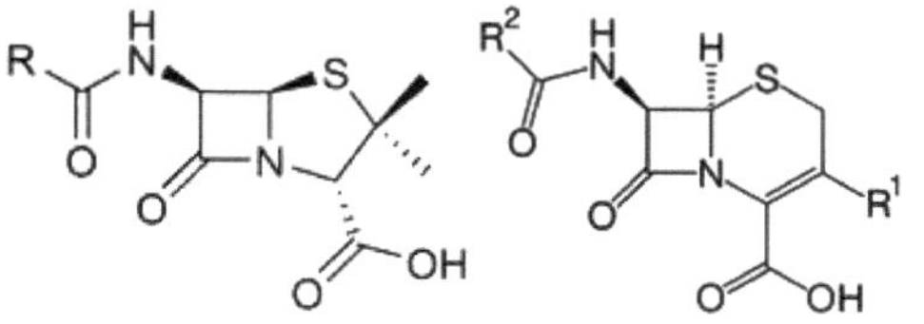

Penicillin molecule Basic nucleus of cephalosporins Figure 2: Chemical structures of beta-lactam sub-groups **(23)**.

4. Aminoglycosides

These antibiotics are reserved for infections that are generally severe. They are active against gram-positive bacteria, particularly staphylococci. They are natural or hemi-synthetic heterosides. They practically do not pass through the wall of the intestine and are therefore less effective. administered by injection, except in the case of local treatment of intestinal infections. Betalactam antibiotics are indicated in the treatment of various infectious diseases, in particular urinary and renal diseases, as they are eliminated in active form by the kidneys. They are : Amikacin, Gentamicin, Netilmicin, Streptomycin, Neomycin, Spectinomycin.

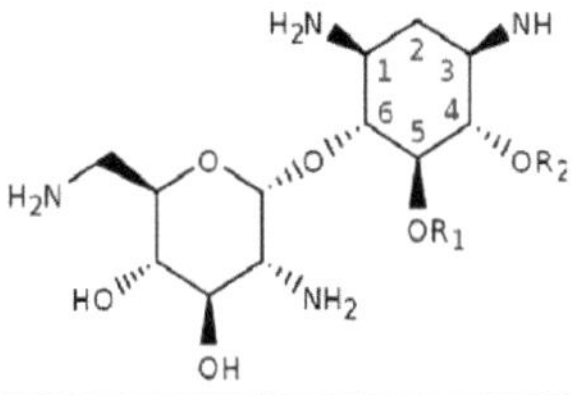

Figure 3: Central nucleus of aminoglycosides (23).

Central core of aminoglycosides, composed of 2-deoxytreptamine (right) and glucosamine (left). This central nucleus corresponds to the antibiotic neamine. The other aminosides are substituted on positions 4 or 5 of deoxystreptamine (positions R1 or R2).

5. Macrolides and related compounds

Macrolides have bacteriostatic or bactericidal activity, depending on their concentration and the sensitivity of the germs. They are effective against aerobic and anaerobic gram-positive cocci, gram-negative cocci such as gonococci and meningococci, gram-negative bacilli such as Helicobacter pylori, and germs such as Legionella pneumophilia, Mycoplasma, Chlamydia and Mycobacterium avium (HIV-infected patients). Some macrolides can be used during pregnancy. Spiramycin is also used in the treatment of toxoplasmosis in pregnant women. These are : Erythromycin, Azithromycin, Clarithromycin, Josamycin, Roxithromycin, Spiramycin, Telithromycin.

6. Lincosamides: Lincomycin

Lincosamines are used in the treatment of a variety of serious infectious diseases, including those of the bronchi, ears, mouth and teeth, skin and bones, and genital tract. They are also used to prevent bacterial endocarditis.

7. Synergistins or streptogramins: Synergistins are mainly used in ENT infections, including acute sinusitis, bronchopulmonary infections, stomatological infections and genital infections (prostatitis),   skin infections bone joint infections. Risk significant of Avoid association with colchicine, ciclosporin or tacrolimus. These are : Pristinamycin quinupristin/dalfopristin

8. Fidaxomicin : Fidaxomicin

Fidaxomicin is bactericidal and inhibits RNA synthesis by bacterial RNA polymerase. It is indicated in adults for the treatment of acute diarrhoea associated with Clostridium difficile. For the moment, this compound is only available in hospitals. The recommended dose is 200 mg (one tablet twice a day for 10 days).

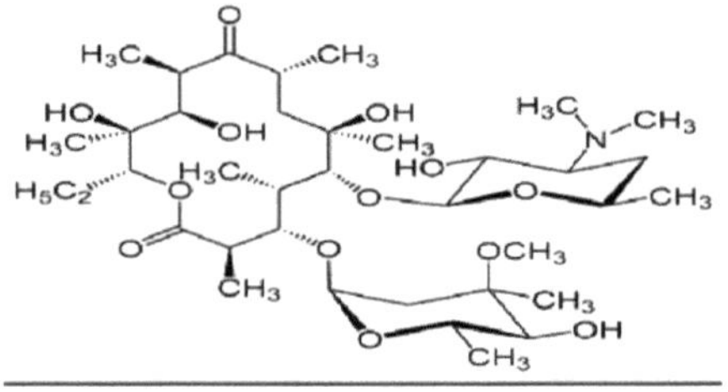

Figure 4: Chemical structure of Erythromycin (23).

9. Quinolones and fluoroquinolones

Quinolones are synthetic antibiotics. They are indicated for genitourinary, gastrointestinal, ENT, osteoarticular, bronchopulmonary, eye and ear infections.

These are : Fluoroquinolones: Norfloxacin, Péfloxacin, Ofloxacin, Lévofloxacin, Ciprofloxacin, Enoxacin, Moxifloxacin, Loméfloxacin.

10. Tetracyclines

Tetracyclines are antibiotics originally isolated from Streptomyces cultures. They are now obtained by hemisynthesis.

These antibiotics are broad-spectrum bacteriostats. They act by inhibiting bacterial protein synthesis. These molecules diffuse well through the tissue.

$1^{\text{ère}}$ **generation cyclins:** Chlortetracycline, Oxytetracycline. These cyclines are only used topically.

$2^{\text{ème}}$ **generation cyclins:** Doxycycline, Minocycline, Limecycline, Methylenecycline,
These cyclins are indicated for acute respiratory tract infections caused by intracellular germs (Chlamydiae, Coxiella, Mycoplasma, etc.), as well as psittacosis and Haemophilus influenzae infections after failure of other treatments. They are indicated in the treatment of acne, periodontitis and Lyme disease. They are the antibiotics of choice for sexually transmitted infections (chlamydia, mycoplasma, syphilis). Doxycycline is used in chemoprophylaxis for malaria.

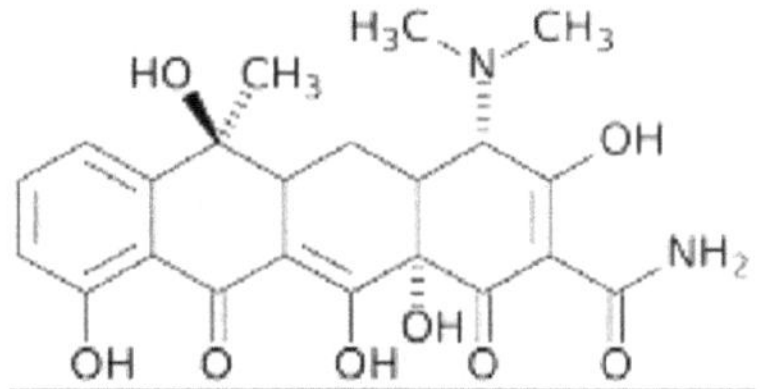

Figure 5: Chemical structure of tetracyclines (23).

11. Glycopeptides

These antibiotics are not absorbed orally and are only used in injectable form. They are indicated in cases of resistant gram-positive infections or allergy to beta-lactam antibiotics. They are: Vancomycin, Teicoplanin.

12. Sulphonamides

They are for

- Local: Sulfadiazine argentique
- ENT: Sulfarazol, in combination with erythromycin, this antibiotic is prescribed for acute otitis media with sensitive germs.
- Intestinal sulphonamides: Sulfasalazine prescribed for haemorrhagic rectocolitis and Crohn's disease.
- Urinary sulphonamides: Sulfamethizol indicated for cystitis.
- General sulphonamides: Sulfadiazine, combination: Sulfamethoxazole + Trimethoprim indicated for pneumoccystis carinii infections, prostatitis, cystitis, otitis, sinusitis, certain bronchopulmonary infections, digestive infections, etc.
- Anti-malarial sulphonamides: Sulfadoxine

Fusidic acid

This antibiotic is bacteriostatic at low doses and bactericidal at higher doses. It is rarely used as monotherapy due to the many resistant strains. It is still mainly indicated for Staphylococcus aureus infections, in combination with to an aminoglycoside or beta-lactam. It is also used as monotherapy in certain cases of bacterial conjunctivitis involving sensitive germs.

Fosfomycin

Fosfomycin is a phosphoric acid derivative. It is injectable and indicated for severe infections in combination with another antibiotic (beta-lactam antibiotics, aminoside, colistin, glycopeptide). Fosfomycin + trometamol is indicated as a single-dose treatment for acute cystitis. These are : Fosfomycin, fosfomycin + trometamol

Linezolid

Antibiotic belonging to the new class of oxazolidinones, indicated in nosocomial infections with gram-positive germs that are resistant or in cases of allergy to other antibiotics. This antibiotic must be initiated in hospital. Example: Linezolid

Polymyxins

This family of antibiotics is active only on Gram-negative germs; these antibiotics are virtually not absorbed by the digestive mucosa. Oral forms are used as intestinal antiseptics. They are still often used in aerosol therapy for pulmonary infections caused by sensitive germs. These are : Polymyxin B, Polymyxin E

Classification according to the mechanism of action of antibiotics

The different classes of antibiotics have different mechanisms of action and most often have several effects on a single bacterium.

Antibiotics that inhibit bacterial wall synthesis

This category includes :

- ß-lactam antibiotics, which inhibit the transpeptidase involved in the synthesis of the
They are only active on growing bacteria that synthesise peptidoglycan.

- Glycopeptides (vancomycin, ristocetin and teicoplanin), which bind to a synthesis intermediate.

- Bacitracin is only active on Gram-positive bacteria. The outer membrane of Gram-negative bacteria is impermeable to this molecule.

Cytoplasmic membrane inhibiting antibiotics

The hydrophobic end of the polymyxins penetrates the membrane and incorporates into the lipid layer, while the hydrophilic end is directed outwards. The result is disorganisation of the membrane structure, leading to cell death.

Antibiotics that inhibit protein synthesis

Prokaryotic ribosomes are not made up of the same proteins as eukaryotic ribosomes, and have different sedimentation coefficients. There are inhibitors of the 50s subunit, which prevent the attachment of a new amino acid to the growing chain (phenicols) or the transfer of the growing chain from the A site to the P site (macrolides, lincosamides, streptogramins); of the 30 Svedberg subunit, which prevent or disrupt the binding of aminoacyl-tRNAs to ribosomes (tetracyclines, aminoglycosides).

Antibiotics active on the metabolism of nucleic acids and their precursors

A distinction is made between antibiotics active on the one hand in the synthesis of RNA and on the other in the synthesis of DNA or its precursors.

- Sulphonamides act on the synthesis of folic acid, a cofactor in the synthesis of purine and pyrimidine bases for incorporation into nucleic acids. Their specific action is due to the fact that eukaryotes do not synthesise folic acid.

- Diamino pyridines inhibit the reduction of folic acid by taking advantage of the difference in sensitivity of bacterial dihydrofolate reductase compared with the enzyme in eukaryotic cells.

Antibiotics that inhibit metabolic pathways

In prokaryotes, metabolism proceeds via a wide variety of pathways because they have acquired the capacity to adapt to life in nutrient environments and survival conditions that are very different from those of eukaryotes. Despite this fact, the number of antibiotic molecules that act at this level and can be used clinically is very small.

Anti-anaerobic antibiotics

Some bacteria are able to live anaerobically using oxygen-independent redox pathways, and can reach redox potential levels that are significantly lower than in eukaryotes. This enables the specific metabolic activation of certain molecules, such as nitroimidazoles, giving them a particular effect on these organisms and other anaerobic parasites.

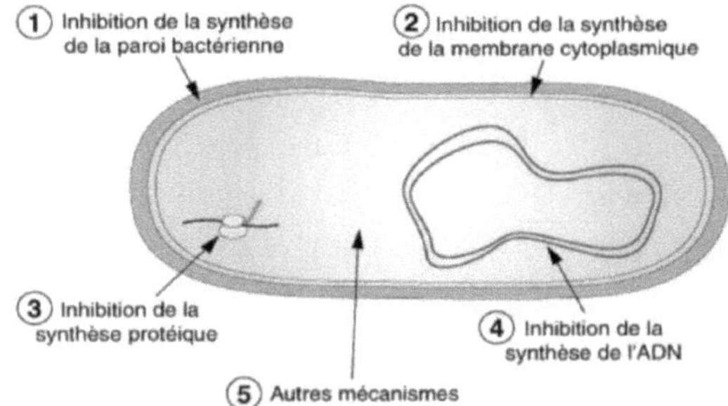

Figure 6: Mechanism of action of antibiotics (24).

Classification of antibiotics according to their spectrum of activity
The spectrum of activity of an antibiotic corresponds to the set of bacterial species that are sensitive to it. A broad-spectrum antibiotic acts on a large

number of bacteria, including gram-positive and gram-positive bacilli and cocci. A narrow-spectrum antibiotic acts only on gram-positive bacilli and cocci (25).

Narrow-spectrum antibiotics: these only kill a limited number of bacteria. They can target and kill the disease-causing bacteria while leaving other bacteria, which may be beneficial, alive.

Broad-spectrum antibiotics: These are effective against many bacteria, including some that are resistant to narrow-spectrum antibiotics(24).

Table I: Classification of antibiotics according to their spectrum(25)

Gram + and Cocci Gram -	Gram bacillus -	Broad spectrum
Penicillin G Penicillin V Anti-staphylococcal Cloxacillin Meticillin in combination with clavulanic acid Lincomycin Clindamycin Macrolides	Ampicillin Amoxicillin Aminoglycoside Polypeptides Furans Quinolones	Sulfonamides / TMP Cephalosporins (variable with generation) Phenicolates Tetracyclines Cotrimoxazole

Good antibiotic prescribing practice Definition of a prescription

In the practice of medicine, prescribing is the act whereby an authorised healthcare professional orders therapeutic recommendations for a patient(26). The steps that every doctor takes to make a diagnosis: the medical history, t h e physical examination and any additional tests.

The first thing a doctor does when he sees you for a consultation is to ask you questions. This is called the history. After asking your age, the doctor will ask you questions in a precise order, from the broadest to the most specific: What are your lifestyle habits? In terms of your profession, where you live, smoking, alcohol, sedentary lifestyle, nutrition, etc.What is your medical history? In terms of illnesses, allergies, operations, disabilities, etc. He or she may ask you whether certain pathologies run in your family. What are your current treatments, whether temporary or chronic? What is the history of your illness? How long have you had symptoms, what are they and how have they developed?

After the medical history, the **physical examination takes place in** 4 stages: **Inspection, which consists of** observing the patient; **palpation**, which consists of touching and palpating certain parts of the body; **percussion, which** looks for abnormal noises by tapping the back of the back, for example; and **auscultation, in which** the doctor listens to certain internal organs (heart, intestines, lungs) with a device called a stethoscope.

Complementary tests are ordered by the doctor if necessary, but not systematically. For example, he may take your blood pressure. Some tests require more equipment. These may include scans, X-rays, MRIs, biopsies, blood tests, etc(27). These may include :

Urine Cytobacteriological Examination (UCE)

The ECBU is a urine examination that detects the possible presence of a pathogenic micro-organism in the urine. This test is essential if a urinary tract infection is suspected. The ECBU is important for detecting any infection of the urogenital sphere. Doctors generally prescribe an ECBU as part of a diagnosis of prostatitis, pyelonephritis **or** cystitis.

ECBU is regularly performed as a screening test in pregnant women to prevent the development of an asymptomatic urinary tract infection. ECBU can also be used to detect a possible infection before an operation or when a urinary catheter is inserted over a long period of time (28).

Analysis of cerebrospinal fluid (CSF)

A CSF test is a series of tests that use a sample of cerebrospinal fluid to help detect brain and spinal cord problems, as well as other conditions affecting the central nervous system. An infection of the brain or spinal cord can cause the following symptoms Severe headache, fever, nausea and vomiting, confusion, sensitivity to light, stiff neck, etc.(29).

Blood culture

Blood culture is a medical test used to detect the presence of pathogenic bacteria or micro-organisms in the blood. It is an essential diagnostic tool for identifying systemic bacterial infections, often referred to as bacteraemia or septicaemia. It is essential that the sample is taken under sterile conditions, to avoid contamination by skin germs, for example, which would distort the results. The sample must also be transported under sterile conditions. Blood cultures may be taken in a number of situations, including suspected septicaemia, prolonged and unexplained fever, complications in people with abscesses, boils or major dental infections, or fever in people with catheters, catheters or prostheses.

Antibiotic susceptibility testing

An antibiotic susceptibility test is a microbiological test which evaluates any acquired resistance of a bacterial strain to the antibiotics to which it is naturally sensitive in the absence of acquired resistance, and which can therefore theoretically be used to treat it. The basic parameter for assessing the sensitivity (or resistance) of a bacterium to an antibiotic is the minimum inhibitory concentration (MIC) of this antibiotic in relation to the bacterium tested (29). The MIC (minimum inhibitory concentration) and the MBC (minimum bactericidal concentration) are required.

An antibiotic can be considered bactericidal when its MBC is approximately equal to its MIC. An antibiotic whose MBC is much higher than the MIC, so that its concentration at the site of infection in vivo does not reach the MBC value, will be considered bacteriostatic(30).

Bacterial resistance to antibiotics.

Antibiotic resistance is the ability of a bacterium to resist the effects of antibiotics. It is one of the forms of drug resistance, different from the phenomenon of antibiotic tolerance (31).

Innate or natural resistance Natural resistance

Natural resistance occurs when all strains of the same bacterial species are resistant to a given antibiotic. Some bacteria are naturally resistant to many molecules. Natural resistance is stable and is passed on to offspring. Its genetic basis is the bacterial chromosome, but it is not, or only to a limited extent, transmissible horizontally, i.e. from one bacterium to another within the same species or between different species. Natural resistance is known and can therefore be circumvented by broadening the spectrum of antibiotics by modifying their chemical structure, as these are in fact bacteria that are insensitive to the antibiotic's mode of action.

Acquired resistance

Acquired resistance occurs when one or more strains of a bacterial species naturally sensitive to an antibiotic become resistant to it. Acquired resistance results from mechanisms linked to the bacterial DNA, and is therefore characterised by mutations or transfers of resistant genes from a resistant bacterium to a susceptible bacterium. The acquisition of resistance genes can result from the transfer of genetic material carrying one or more resistance genes from a resistant bacterium. This second mechanism is the most widespread and the most worrying, as it may simultaneously involve several antibiotics, or even several families of antibiotics. The same bacterial strain can accumulate resistance mechanisms, mutations or gene acquisition, giving rise to multi-resistance. Multi-resistant bacteria or MRB, resistant to several families of antibiotics, and pan-resistant bacteria are those that lead to therapeutic impasses. It is not the antibiotics that cause mutations; mutations are a rare but natural phenomenon. However, the presence of antibiotics tends to favour the resistant strain: antibiotics eliminate non-mutated bacteria, while mutated bacteria resist and can multiply, rendering antibiotic treatment ineffective.

Resistance mechanisms

Inactivation of antibiotics by the production of specific enzymes.

The enzymes produced by the bacteria disorganise and break the specific bonds between the antibiotic and its target, leading to its ineffectiveness. Betalactamases, enzymes produced by bacteria, degrade antibiotics of the Betalactam class, which act by inhibiting peptidoglycan synthesis. Extended-spectrum beta-lactamases (ESBLs) are a large, highly heterogeneous family of bacterial enzymes discovered in the 1980s in France, which give bacteria the ability to hydrolyse a wide variety of penicillins, as well as cephalosporins.

Impermeability of the bacteria to antibiotics.

By varying the permeability of the cytoplasmic membrane, the bacterium prevents the antibiotic from penetrating the cytoplasm.

Elimination of antibiotics by efflux pumps.

The synthesis or acquisition of efflux pumps by the bacteria prevents the antibiotic from accumulating in the intracellular environment. Concentration levels are then insufficient to cause the death of the bacteria. Several classes of antibiotics are involved, including tetracyclines, fluoroquinolones and aminoglycosides.

Modification of the target.

Bacteria modify the conformation of the target or prevent the antibiotic from binding to its site of action by camouflaging the target sites. In this way, even at high concentrations, the antibiotic remains intact and active but has no effect(32).

Another mechanism: "altruism

In addition to these very well described mechanisms, highly resistant bacteria are capable of synthesising indole in very large quantities to meet the needs of sensitive bacteria. Only a minority of highly resistant individuals stand out, these mutants helping the others by producing indole, which helps the cells to fight oxidative stress and get rid of antibiotics. This prevents the weakest cells from dying and gives them time to acquire resistance in their turn. This organic compound has a dual resistance function: efflux of antibiotics and activation of a metabolic pathway (33).

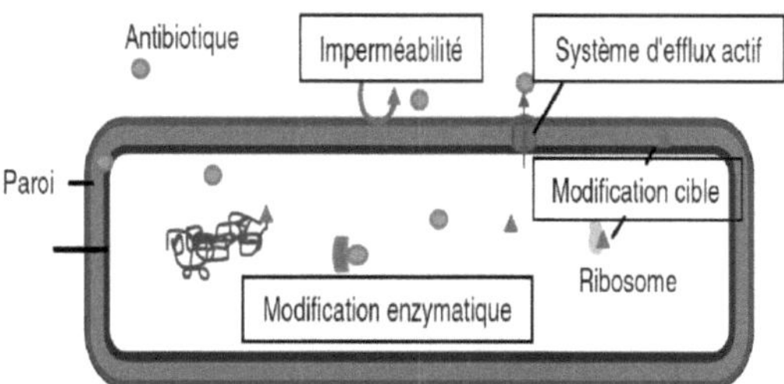

Figure 7: Resistance mechanism (34).

Indication for antibiotic therapy (35) .

Antibiotics are prescribed to combat certain bacterial infections. But what precautions should be taken when using these medicines? By going into these details, we will set out the practical rules for using antibiotics.

Practical rules for the use of antibiotics :

Curative antibiotic therapy

Curative antibiotic therapy is antibiotic therapy designed to treat a progressive infection.

It can be adapted to a particular bacterium from the outset, when the infection has been documented and antibiotic sensitivity is known from an antibiogram. It can also be probabilistic, i.e. prescribed before knowing the bacteria involved and/or their sensitivity to the antibiotic. It is a reasoned prescription, taking into account the bacteria usually responsible for a given infection and their usual sensitivity to the various antibiotics administered for these indications.

Prophylactic or preventive antibiotic therapy

Prophylactic antibiotic therapy is antibiotic therapy prescribed to prevent the development of a specific infection under certain conditions. It is also given before surgery, as it is known that opening the skin can lead to infection. An injection of antibiotic is therefore given 30 minutes before the incision is made.

Antibiotic monotherapy or dual therapy

In the majority of cases, infections in towns and cities are treated with a **monotherapy**. There is no indication for a combination. On the other hand, in people hospitalised with an infection presenting more severe clinical pictures with slightly more resistant bacteria, dual therapy may be introduced. Combination therapy can also be prescribed for people who regularly take antibiotics and who are at risk of developing antibiotic-resistant bacteria.

Duration of antibiotic therapy

Antibiotic therapy may be prescribed for a period ranging from a few days to several weeks or even months. The duration of antibiotic treatment depends on the source of the infection. For serious infections, prolonged antibiotic treatment can last up to 6 to 12 weeks.

Monitoring antibiotic therapy

Antibiotic therapy is monitored primarily for the risk of allergy. This is why the question of allergy to antibiotics, particularly those in the penicillin or cephalosporin family, should always be raised before starting antibiotic treatment. It is also important to warn patients of the frequent side effects and to tell them how to take the antibiotics to limit these effects. For prolonged courses of antibiotics, beyond 7 days, biological tests are carried out every 7 to 10 days, particularly for antibiotics that may be toxic to the liver or kidneys.

Combination of antibiotics :

When deciding on antibiotic therapy, a combination of antibiotics may be chosen for three main reasons:

- A broader antibacterial spectrum;
- Preventing the selection of resistant germs;
- Increased bactericidal speed through synergistic action.
In bacteriology, antibiotic combinations are characterised by interactions:

- Indifference: the activity of one antibiotic is not affected by the presence of the other;
- Addition: the effect of the combination is equal to the sum of the effects of each antibiotic studied separately at the same concentration as in the combination;

- synergy: the effect of the combination is significantly greater than the sum of the activities of each antibiotic studied separately (36).

The rules established by Jawetz and Gunnison in 1952 still provide a sound rationale for treatment, although more recent studies specific to each antibiotic may put these data into perspective. These rules are based on the following principle: if a bacteriostatic antibiotic prevents germs from multiplying by its mode of action, it reduces the proportion of germs in the multiplication phase and therefore the efficacy of a bactericidal antibiotic, which is active on multiplying germs. Thus :

- The combination of two bactericidal antibiotics can produce a synergistic effect.
- The combination of two bacteriostatic antibiotics generally has an additive effect.
- Combining a bactericidal antibiotic with a bacteriostatic antibiotic can have an antagonistic effect(37).

METHODOLOGICAL APPROACH

A cross-sectional, descriptive study was carried out in paediatric services in the Bamako district, involving two hospitals, Mali Hospital and Gabriel Touré Hospital, two reference health centres (Commune V and Commune VI) and two CSCOMs (Yirimadio and Kalaban Coura). It took place over three months, from April 2023 to June 2023.

Data were collected from prescriptions and registers as primary sources of information, and from children under five (5) years of age and prescribers as secondary sources. Using a reasoned choice approach, 481 prescriptions were selected and all prescribers who had issued the sampled prescriptions were interviewed.

All children under 5 years of age seen in paediatric wards at the 6 study sites who had been prescribed antibiotics and whose parents agreed to take part in the study were included in our study.

The study focused on the dependent variable represented by the quality of the prescription, and the other independent variables concerned the prescriber, the prescribing site, the patient, the diagnosis, the indications for antibiotic therapy, the antibiotic used and the prescription (see table below).

Data was entered using Microsoft Word 2016, and analysed using SPSS and Excel. The statistical tests used were Pearson's Chi-square or, failing that, Fisher's exact test, with a 95% confidence interval.

From an ethical point of view, a letter of introduction was deposited in each institution and the agreement of the staff working in the department was obtained before each collection. All our patients were given an anonymity number. Only this number was used for data entry and analysis. No patient was included in our study without prior explicit consent. Our data were only used to improve prescribing and patient management. In the event of dissemination, through a presentation in a scientific forum or publication in a scientific journal, the identity of the patients will not be known.

Study variables

Dependent variable	Independent variables	Characteristic of independent variables
	Prescriber and prescription site	- Number of years' experience of prescriber, - Site of prescription, - Gender Profile, - Training received on antibiotic therapy, - RENAM available.
	Patient	- Entry date; Age, - Gender, - Parents' occupations, Allergy(ies), - Inpatient or outpatient, Reason for - hospitalisation, - Child's weight,
Prescription quality	Diagnosis and indications for antibiotic therapy	- Germ(s), Pathology(ies) involved Nature - of sample, - Availability of antibiograms
	Antibiotic therapy	- Antibiotic family, Antibiotic name, Route - of administration, Dosage - Number of times daily, Side effects
	Prescription and prescription	- Patient's surname and first name(s) ; - Prescriber's name ; - Prescriber's address ; - Presence of the patient's age ; - Prescriber's signature ; - Sex of patient mentioned ; - Prescriber's stamp ; - Patient's weight ; - Date of prescription mentioned.

Operationalisation of the main variable

- According to our method, a prescription is of good quality when it meets the following requirements:

- The diagnosis is consistent with the drug prescribed according to the RENAM or other national recommendation,

- Dosage is in accordance with RENAM recommendations or other national recommendations,

- The dosage is in accordance with the requirements of the RENAM or other national recommendation,

- The duration of treatment is in accordance with the RENAM or other national recommendations,

- Galenic form respected,

- The route of administration is in accordance with the indications in the RENAM or other national recommendations.

- However, if a prescription does not meet all of these requirements, it is deemed to be of insufficient quality according to our criteria.

RESULTS

During the period of our study, we collected 481 prescriptions for antibiotics. The information gathered from the prescriptions and the registers gave us the following results

Socio-demographic characteristics of children prescribed antibiotics

Table II: Breakdown of patients by socio-demographic characteristics of study targets

Socio-demographic characteristics	Variables	Number of employees (%)	95% CI
	[0-12]	243 (50,5)	46,07-54,97
Age range	[12-59]	238 (49,5)	42,21-57,55
	Female	221 (46,0)	41,75-50,62
Gender	Male	260 (54,0)	49,38-58,25
	Bamako	19 (4,0)	2,71-6,33
Region of origin	Outside Bamako	452 (94,0)	91,24-99,5
	Outside Mali	10 (2,0)	1,13-3,78
	Community health centre	276 (57,4)	52,92-61,72
Prescription site	Reference centre	145 (30,1)	26,22-34,39
	Hospital	60 (12,5)	9,82-15,73

The age range [0-12] accounted for 50.5% of cases. The mean age was 17.7 months, with extremes of 1 and 59 months. Males predominated, accounting for 54% of cases. The sex ratio was 1.17. The majority of cases came from outside Bamako (94%). The CSCOMs were in the majority, accounting for 57.4% of cases.

Socio-demographic characteristics of parents of children prescribed antibiotics

Table III: Breakdown of patients by parental characteristics

Features of parents	Variable	Workforce	Percentage	95% CI
	Primary	34	7,2	5,1-9,72
	Secondary	106	22,1	18,56-25,96
	Superior	125	26,1	22,27-30,09
Level of education of	Koranic school	105	21,8	18,37-25,74
Fathers	No	79	16,4	13,38-20,0
	Not specified	32	6,4	4,75-9,24
	Retailer	144	29,9	26,02-34,18
	Employee	106	22	18,56-25,96
Fathers' occupations	Worker	102	21,2	17,79-25,08
	Civil servant	60	12,5	9,82-15,73
	Farmer	18	3,8	2,38-5,84
	Student	1	0,2	0,04-1,17
	Not specified	27	5,6	3,89-8,04
	Not enrolled	201	41,8	37,46-46,24
	Primary	38	7,9	5,81-10,66
Level of education of	Secondary	90	18,7	15,48-22,44
Mothers	Superior	75	15,6	12,62-19,11
	Koranic school	74	15,4	12,44-18,88
	Not specified	3	0,6	0,21-1,82
	Housekeeper	313	65,1	60,71-69,2
	Retailer	94	19,5	16,25-23,32
	Employee	27	5,6	3,89-8,04
Mothers' occupations	Civil servant	23	4,8	3,21-7,07
	Pupil/Student	22	4,6	3,04-6,83
	Not specified	1	0,4	0,04-1,17
	Others to be specified	1	0,4	0,04-1,17

Shopkeepers represented 29.9% of our sample for fathers and housewives represented 65.1% for mothers. Higher education represented 26.1% of cases for fathers and 41.8% for mothers.

Characteristics of prescribers

Table IV: Breakdown of prescribers by prescriber characteristics

Characteristics of specifiers	Variables	Workforce n=25	Percentage	95% CI
	Male	17	68	46,5-85,05
Gender	Female	8	32	14,95-53,50
	General practitioner	7	28	12,07-49,39
Profile	Internal	13	52	31,31-72,20
	Paediatrician	2	8	0,98-26,03
	DES in paediatrics	3	12	2,55-31,22
Number of years	> 03 years	16	64	50,06-80,02
Experience	≤ 03 years	9	36	20,8-50,9
Training received	Yes	5	20	15,68-31,64
	No	20	80	72,49-93,85
Availability of	No	24	96	79,65-99,9
RENAM	Yes	2	8	5,45-10,19
Total		25	100,0	

Males accounted for 68% of cases. Sex ratio (M/F): 2.12. Residents accounted for 52% of cases. The majority of prescribers had more than 03 years' experience, i.e. 64% of cases. 20% of prescribers had received training in antibiotic therapy. RENAM was available to 4% of prescribers

State of health of children prescribed antibiotics Children's medical history

Table V: Distribution of patients according to clinical characteristics.

Features clinics	Variable	Workforce	Percentage	95% CI
Status at birth	Term	476	99	98,18-99,79
	No term	5	1	0,21-1,82
	Correct	461	95,8	93,67-97,29
Vaccination status	Incomplete	12	2,5	1,43-4,31
	Not done	8	1,7	0,85-3,25
	Age-appropriate	435	90,4	87,48-92,61
Power supply	Not suitable	37	7,7	5,63-10,42
	Not specified	9	1,9	0,99-3,52
Allergy	Yes	28	5,8	4,06-8,28
	No	453	94,2	91,72-95,94
	Ambulatory	442	92,0	89,81-94,55
Tracking mode	Hospitalized	39	8,0	5,45-10,19

The majority of births were at term (99% of cases). Vaccination was correct in 95.8% of cases. Diet was appropriate for the age of the child in 90.4% of cases. Allergies were present in 5.8% of patients. The main symptoms of these allergies were sneezing, runny nose, coughing, skin rash and itching. 92% of the children were outpatients.

The condition of children on admission to healthcare facilities

Table VI: Distribution of patients according to signs of onset of the disease

Signs of the onset of the disease	Number n=481	Percentage	95% CI	
Fever	338	70,3	67,03-73,64	
Rhinorrhea	182	35,1	31,9-39,04	
Cough	169	37,8	32,08-42,89	
Diarrhoea	95	19,7	16,07-20,03	
Vomiting	65	13,5	9,05-18,7	
Skin rash	54	11,2	8,6-14,9	
Headache	25	5,2	2,4-9,01	
Convulsion	9	1,9	0,99-3,52	
Other	14	2,9	1,74-4,83	

Other: anorexia (8), asthenia (4), swelling (2)

Fever was the main sign of onset, accounting for 70.3% of cases.

Table VII: Breakdown of patients by condition on admission

Condition on admission	Variable	Workforce	Percentage	95% CI
	36	59	12,3	9,63-15,5
	37	194	40,3	36,04-44,78
Temperature	38	178	37,0	32,81-41,41
	39	42	8,7	6,55-11,59
	40	8	1,7	0,85-3,25
	Altered	31	6,5	4,58-9,00
General condition	Good	345	71,7	67,54-75,57
	Fair	105	21,8	18,37-25,74
	MAM	10	2,1	1,13-3,78
Nutritional status	MAS	14	2,9	1,74-4,83
	Normal	457	95	92,68-96,62

The most common temperature was 37°C, accounting for 40.3% of cases. The mean was 37.5°C, with extremes of 36.0 and 40.0°C. General condition was good in 71.7% of cases. MAM accounted for 2.1% of cases.

Table VIII: Distribution of patients according to physical signs of infection

Physical sign		Number n=481	Percentage	95% CI
Isolated fever		120	24,9	21,04-28,01
Digestive		93	19,3	16,1-23,01
Pulmonary		82	17,0	14,1-20,0
Cutaneous		68	14,1	10,6-17,09
ENT		53	11,1	8,97-14,01
Neurological		7	1,5	0,57-2,69
Urinary		2	0,4	0,11-1,5
Not specified	51	10,6	7,1-14,01	

Isolated fever was the main physical sign, accounting for 24.9% of cases.

Table IX: Breakdown of patients according to the diagnostic hypotheses evoked

Assumptions	Number n=481	Percentage	95% CI	
Respiratory infections	291	60,4	56,3-65,01	
Malaria	65	13,5	8,54-17,87	
Gastroenteritis	51	10,6	6,89-14,01	
Varicella	38	7,9	3,83-10,07	
Meningitis	17	3,5	1,5-7,43	
Allergy	4	0,8	0,32-2,12	
Wound infection	4	0,8	0,32-2,12	
Abscess	3	0,6	0,21-1,82	
Conjunctivitis	3	0,6	0,21-1,82	
Candidiasis	3	0,6	0,21-1,82	
Otitis	2	0,4	0,11-1,5	
Burn	1	0,2	0,04-1,82	

Respiratory infection was the most common hypothesis (60.4%).

Secondary diagnostic tests Table X: Biological tests

Examination biological	Variable	Workforce	Percentage	95% CI
	Not done	426	88,5	85,18-90,92
	Normal	23	4,8	3,21-7,07
NFS	Hyperleukocytosis with PNN	20	4,2	2,71-6,33
	Thrombocytopenia	8	1,7	0,85-3,25
	Lymphocytic hyperleukocytosis	4	0,8	0,32-2,12
	Positive	14	2,9	1,74-4,83
CRP	Negative	19	4,0	2,54-6,09
	Not done	448	93,1	90,52-95,07
	Positive	4	0,8	0,32-2,12
CSF ECB	Negative	2	0,4	0,11-1,5
	Not done	475	98,6	97,03-99,29
	Positive	18	3,7	2,38-5,84
TDR/GE	Negative	171	35,6	31,40-39,93
	Not done	292	60,7	56,27-64,97

Hyperleukocytosis with PNN accounted for 4.2% of cases. CRP was positive in 2.9% of cases. Positive ECB represented 0.8% of cases. RDT/GE was positive in 18 patients, a rate of 3.7%.

Table XI: Distribution of patients according to radiography.

Radiography	Workforce n=481	Percentage	95% CI
Normal	3	0,6	0,21-4,78
Pathological	23	4,8	3,21-7,07
Not done	455	94,6	92,20-96,28
Total	481	100,0	

X-rays were pathological in 4.8% of cases.

Table XII: Breakdown of patients by diagnosis

Diagnostics	Number n=481	Percentage	95% CI
Respiratory infections	146	30,3	26,04-34,76
Tonsillitis	69	14,3	10,2-19,91
Malaria	56	11,6	9,05-17,87
ENT infection	52	10,9	8,1-15,87
Rhinobronchitis	47	9,8	6,99-14,6
Amoebiasis	18	3,7	2,35-6,09
Candidiasis	17	3,6	2,18-5,89
Malnutrition and fever	15	3,1	2,08-5,78
Pyoderma	13	2,8	1,59-4,57
Varicella	12	2,6	1,02-3,98
Conjunctivitis	8	1,7	0,85-3,25
Meningitis	4	0,8	0,32-2,12
Epilepsy	4	0,8	0,32-2,12
Heart disease and fever	4	0,8	0,32-2,12
Dehydration and fever	3	0,6	0,21-1,82
Allergy	3	0,6	0,21-1,82
Periodontitis	3	0,6	0,21-1,82
Paracetamol poisoning	2	0,4	0,11-1,50
Other	5	1,0	0,21-1,82
Total	481	100,0	

Other: Genital infection, Urinary infection, Ionic disorder, Circumcision, Thermal burns

Respiratory infection was the most frequently mentioned diagnosis (30.3%).

Table XIII: Breakdown of patients by reason for hospitalisation

Reason for hospitalisation	Number n=37	Percentage	95% CI	
Respiratory distress	18	48,6	42,04-52,03	
Convulsion	10	27,2	24,8-31,09	
Dehydration	2	5,4	1,67-9,83	
MAS	2	5,4	1,67-9,83	
Abdominal pain	1	2,7	0,99-3,67	
Drop	1	2,7	0,99-3,67	
Undernutrition	1	2,7	0,99-3,67	
Pneumonia	1	2,7	0,99-3,67	

Respiratory distress was the main reason for hospitalisation, accounting for 48.6% of cases.

Prescribing antibiotics

Table XIV: Breakdown of patients by antibiotics prescribed

Antibiotics	Number n=481	Percentage	95% CI
Ceftriaxone	181	37,6	33,49-41,09
Amoxicillin	135	28,0	24,81-32,09
Gentamycin	104	21,6	18,67-25,01
Erythromycin	51	10,6	7,01-14,02
Cefixime	47	9,8	6,01-13,69
Amoxicillin + clavulanic acid	42	8,7	5,2-12,03
Metronidazole	35	7,2	4,02-11,89
Azytromicin	16	3,3	1,02-6,45
Cotrimoxazole	6	1,2	0,57-2,69
Doxycycline	5	1,0	0,45-2,42
Polymicin B	2	0,4	0,11-1,50
Other	3	0,6	0,21-1,82

Others: Vancomycin, Norfloxacin, Flucoxacillin

Ceftriaxone was the most prescribed antibiotic, appearing on 37.6% of prescriptions.

Table XV: Breakdown of patients by antibiotic family prescribed.

Family	Number n=481	Percentage	95% CI
Betalactam antibiotics	389	80,9	73,01-84,86
Aminosides	107	22,2	18,82-26,09
Macrolides	64	13,3	9,67-16,98
Nitro imidazoles	35	7,2	4,31-10,89
Tetracyclines	7	1,4	0,88-3,47
Sulfonamides	5	1,0	0,45-2,42
Fluoroquinolones	3	0,6	0,21-1,82
Polypeptides	1	0,2	0,04-1,17
Glycopeptide	1	0,2	0,04-1,17

The beta-lactam family was the most prescribed, accounting for 80.9% of cases.

Table XVI: Breakdown of patients by dosage of antibiotics prescribed per prescription

Dosage	Variable	Workforce n=481	%	95% CI
	Single antibiotic therapy	347	72,14	65,4-75,59
Number	Bi antibiotic therapy	125	25,98	24,63-32,67
	Tri-antibiotic therapy	9	1,88	0,99-3,52
Route of administration	Oral	263	54,6	50,21-59,07
	Parenteral	204	42,4	38,07-46,87
	Local	14	2,91	1,74-4,83
	Short	264	54,9	50,42-59,28
Duration	Long	138	28,7	24,83-32,89
	Not specified	79	16,4	13,38-20,00
	Twice	280	58,21	53,76-62,54
Number of catches perday	Once	195	40,54	36,24-44,99
	Three times	6	1,26	0,57-2,69

Single antibiotic therapy was used in the majority of cases (72.14%). Local route: cutaneous, auricular and ocular application. The oral route accounted for 54.6% of cases. Short: less than or equal to 7 days; Long: more than 7 days. The duration of antibiotic therapy was short in 264 patients, i.e. 54.9% of cases.

Twice-daily administration accounted for 58.21% of cases.

Table XVII: Breakdown by antibiotic combination

Types of association	Workforce n=481	Percentage	95% CI
No association	347	72,2	65,4-75,59
Ceftriaxone + gentamycin	90	18,8	15,1-22,87
Amoxicillin + metronidazole	5	1,1	0,45-2,42
Erythromycin + metronidazole	5	1,1	0,45-2,42
Amoxicillin + ceftriaxone	4	0,8	0,32-2,12
Amoxicillin + azithromycin	4	0,8	0,32-2,12
Cefixime + metronidazole	4	0,8	0,32-2,12
Erythromycin + gentamycin	4	0,8	0,32-2,12
Amoxicillin + tetracycline	3	0,6	0,21-1,82
Metronidazole + cotrimoxazole	2	0,4	1,67-9,83
Metronidazole + norfloxazole	2	0,4	1,67-9,83
Amoxi +clavunic acid +gentamycin	1	0,2	0,04-1,17
Tetracycline + gentamicin	1	0,2	0,04-1,17
Ceftriaxone +gentamycin +Amoxicillin	1	0,2	0,04-1,17
Ceftriaxone + vancomycin	1	0,2	0,04-1,17
Cefixime+ amoxicillin	1	0,2	0,04-1,17
Ceftriaxone +gentamycin +erythromycin	3	0,2	0,21-1,82
Erythromycin + tetracycline	1	0,2	0,04-1,17
Gentamycin + amoxicillin	1	0,2	0,04-1,17
Metronidazole +tetracycline	1	0,2	0,04-1,17
Penicillin G + gentamycin	1	0,2	0,04-1,17
Tetracycline + gentamycin	1	0,2	0,04-1,17
Total	481	100,0	

The ceftriaxone + gentamycin combination accounted for 18.8% of cases.

Motivation for prescribing antibiotics to children in the study Table XVIII: Distribution of patients according to the reason for prescribing.

Justification	Workforce n=481	Percentage	95% CI
Infectious hypothesis	476	99,0	97,59-99,59
Confirmed infection	3	0,6	0,21-1,82
Systematic in malnourished patients	2	0,4	0,11-1,50
Total	481	100,0	

Confirmed infections were present in 3 patients, representing a rate of 0.6% of cases. **Compliance of antibiotic prescriptions with diagnoses according t o national guidelines**

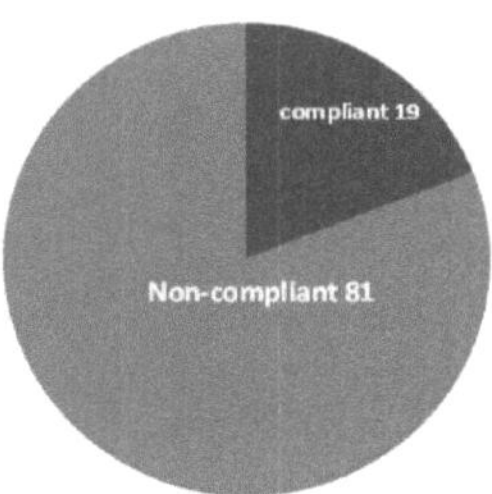

Figure 8: Distribution according to compliance with RENAM or other national standards

Antibiotic prescribing was compliant with the national prescribing guidelines in only 19% of cases (95% CI: [16.05-23.10], but non-compliant in 81% (95% CI: [76.90-83.95]).

Factors influencing the quality of prescriptions

Table XIX: Prescribing quality by prescriber profile

		Compliant	
Profile of Prescriber	Yes (%)	No (%)	Total (%)
Doctor general practitioner	5 (41,6)	2 (15,4)	7 (28,0)
Internal	3 (25,0)	10 (77,0)	13 (52,0)
Paediatrician	4 (33,33)	1 (7,6)	5 (20,0)
Total	12 (100)	13 (100)	25 (100)

Fischer=7.38 p=0.081 (p>0.05)

GPs prescribed 41.6% of the drugs, followed by interns 25%. The difference was not statistically significant (p>0.05).

Table XX: Prescribing quality according to the number of years' experience of the prescriber

Years of experience	Compliant			Total (%)
	Yes (%)	No (%)		
≤ 3 years	2 (28,6)	7 (38,9)		9 (36,0)
> 3 years	5 (71,4)	11 (61,1)		16 (64,0)
Total	7 (100)	18 (100)		25 (100)

Fischer=1.996 p=0.383 (p>0.05) 95% CI: 0.349-1.161

28.6% of prescribers with ≤ 3 years' experience and 71.4% of prescribers with > 3 years' experience prescribed in accordance with RENAM or another national reference. The difference was not statistically significant (p>0.05).

Table XXI: Prescribing quality according to antibiotic therapy training received

Training received on antibiotic therapy	Compliant		Total (%)
	Yes (%)	No (%)	
Yes	4 (33,33)	1 (7,7)	5 (20,0)
No	8 (66,67)	12 (92,30)	20 (80,0)
Total	12 (100)	13 (100)	25 (100)

Fischer=6.782 p=0.029 (p<0.05) 95% CI: 0.242-5.616

Prescribers who had received training in antibiotic therapy prescribed 33.33% compliant prescriptions. The difference is statistically significant (p<0.05).

Table XXII: Prescription quality according to the availability of RENAM

Availability of the document RENAM	Compliant		Total (%)
	Yes (%)	No (%)	
Yes	1 (12,5)	1 (5,9)	2 (8)
No	7 (87,5)	16 (94,1)	23 (92)
Total	8 (100)	17 (100)	25 (100)

Fischer=2,224 p =0.148 (p>0.05) 95% CI: 1.341-2.984

12.5% of prescribers who had access to the RENAM prescribed compliant prescriptions. The difference was not statistically significant p>0.05.

Table XXIII: Prescription quality by sex of child

		Compliant	
Child's gender	Yes (%)	No (%)	Total (%)
Male	46 (51,7)	176 (44,9)	222 (46,1)
Female	43 (48,3)	216 (55,1)	259 (53,9)
Total	89 (100)	392 (100)	481 (100)

Chi2=1.345 ddl=1 p=0,246 (p>0,05)

Of the male children, 51.7% received compliant prescriptions. The difference was not statistically significant (p>0.05).

Table XXIV: Prescribing quality by sex of prescriber

		Compliant	
Sex of prescriber	Yes (%)	No (%)	Total (%)
Male	5 (71,4)	12 (66,7)	17 (68,0)
Female	2 (28,6)	6 (33,3)	8 (32,0)
Total	7 (100)	18 (100)	25 (100)

Fischer=0.063 p=0.83 (p>0.05)

Prescribing conformed to the RENAM for 71.4% of male prescribers and 28.6% of female prescribers. The difference was not statistically significant p >0.05.

Table XXV: Quality of prescriptions by age group of child

Compliant			
Age range from the child	Yes (%)	No (%)	Total (%)
[0- 12] months	48 (53,9)	195 (49,7)	243 (50,5)
[13-59] months	41 (46,1)	197 (50,3)	238 (49,5)
Total	89 (100)	392 (100)	481 (100)

p=0.476 (p>0.05)

In the [0-12] months age group, 48% of prescriptions were compliant, and in the [13-59] months age group, 41% were compliant. The difference was not statistically significant (P>0.05).

Table XXVI: Quality of prescriptions by father's profession

Compliant			
Professionof fathers	Yes (%)	No (%)	Total (%)
Retailer	29 (32,6)	115 (29,3)	144 (29,9)
Civil servant	12 (13,5)	48 (12,2)	60 (12,5)
Not specified	4 (4,4)	23 (5,9)	27 (5,6)
Worker	7 (7,8)	95 (24,2)	102 (21,2)
Farmer	7 (7,8)	11 (2,8)	18 (3,7)
Non-civil servant	23 (25,8)	83 (21,2)	106 (22,1)
Others to be specified	7 (7,8)	17 (4,1)	23 (4,8)
Total	89 (100)	392 (100)	481 (100)

p=0.008 (p< 0.05)

Children whose fathers were shopkeepers received 29% compliant prescriptions, followed by 23% for salaried employees and 12% for civil servants. The difference is statistically significant, p<0.05.

Table XXVII: Prescription quality by monitoring mode

		Compliant	
Tracking mode	Yes (%)	No (%)	Total (%)
Ambulatory	76 (85,3)	369 (94,1)	445 (92,5)
Hospitalized	13 (14,7)	23 (5,9)	36 (7,5)
Total	89 (100)	392 (100)	481 (100)

p=0.005 (P<0.05)

Outpatients received 76% compliant prescriptions. The difference was statistically significant at P<0.05.

Table XXVIII: Quality of prescriptions according to the diagnosis used

Compliant				
Diagnosis selected	Yes (%)		No (%)	Total (%)
Respiratory infections	26 (29,2)		120 (30,6)	146 (30,3)
Tonsillitis		5 (5,7)	64 (16,3)	69 (14,3)
Malaria		2 (2,3)	54 (13,8)	56 (11,6)
ENT infection		2 (2,3)	50 (12,7)	52 (10,9)
Rhinobronchitis		1 (1,1)	46 (11,7)	47 (9,8)
Amoebiasis		8 (9,0)	10 (2,5)	18 (3,7)
Candidiasis		7 (7,6)	10 (2,5)	17 (3,6)
Malnutrition and fever		5 (5,4)	10 (2,5)	15 (3,1)
Pyoderma		8 (9,0)	5 (1,2)	13 (2,8)
Varicella		8 (9,0)	4 (1,0)	12 (2,6)
Epilepsy		2 (2,2)	2 (0,5)	4 (0,8)
Heart disease and fever		2 (2,2)	2 (0,5)	4 (0,8)
Dehydration and fever		1 (1,1)	2 (0,5)	3 (0,6)
Other		12(13,5)	13(3,3)	25 (5,2)
Total	89 (100)		392 (100)	481 (100)

Patients with respiratory infections received 29.2% compliant prescriptions. But for all prescriptions in relation to the pathologies diagnosed, compliance in terms of antibiotic prescribing was only 19%, with non-compliance accounting for 81%.

<h1 style="text-align:center">COMMENTS AND DISCUSSIONS</h1>

In terms of achieving the objectives, the aim of this study was to evaluate the quality of antibiotic prescribing in six (06) health services in Bamako in 2023. In the end, we achieved our objectives, but certain constraints limited the study. We did not take into account all antibiotic prescriptions because they were made in several consultation rooms at the various study sites. Time and human resources did not allow us to be exhaustive in this respect. In addition, we noted that RENAM had not given precise directives concerning certain diagnoses, which did not favour the harmonisation of prescriptions in relation to the same diagnosis. However, this did not call into question the validity of the data observed.

With regard to the characteristics of the subjects of the study, in relation to the age and sex of the children, out of 481 prescriptions collected, 54% were male, with a sex ratio of 1.17. The same finding was made by Bamba A Sangaré (8) in 2020, with a sex ratio of 1.3. The same finding was made by Bamba A Sangaré (8) in 2020, with a sex ratio of 1.3. Hiddou et al (12) in 2018 obtained a sex ratio of 1.07. This could be explained in part by the fact that at this age of development, the male sex is more active and more turbulent, which exposes it to many health problems. The [0-12] months age group was the most represented with 50.5%, the average age was 17.7 months with extremes of 1 and 59 months.

In terms of prescribers, 68% of prescriptions were written by male prescribers, with a sex ratio of 2.12. This result is contrary to the study by Camille A in 2020 (40), which found that 54.7% of prescriptions were written by women. This result is contrary to the study conducted by Camille A in 2020 (40), which found that 54.7% of prescriptions were written by women. The majority of prescribers (64%) had been prescribing for more than 3 years. This could be explained by the fact that most prescribers were general practitioners, interns or paediatricians with several years' experience.The majority of prescriptions (52%) were prescribed by internists and 28% by general practitioners. These results are contrary to those found by Sellam et al (38) in 2015, who obtained 21% of prescriptions by general practitioners and 12% by paediatricians, and by Adissa et al (39) in 2018 after a similar study carried out in south-west Nigeria, with a result of 48.5% of prescriptions by doctors. They are also contrary to those found by Ciré et al (40) on the "Prescription of antibiotics in the paediatric ward of the Ignace Deen National Hospital in Conakry in 2020", with 55% of prescriptions by general practitioners and 45% by specialists.

In terms of prescriptions issued, almost all the prescriptions we received included the patient's name. This can be explained by the fact that most prescriptions include a heading for the patient's name. Age and sex were given in 97.1% and 94.4% of the prescriptions in our sample respectively. Weight was mentioned in 79.4% of our samples, which can be explained by the fact that, in paediatric wards, children's weights are taken systematically on arrival, and that this enables the dosage of antibiotics to be adjusted in children. The majority of our sample was collected in ComHCs (57.4%), followed by 30.1% collected in CSREFs and 12.5% in hospitals. This high prescription rate in ComHCs can be explained by the fact that ComHCs are the first point of contact with patients before being referred to other levels of the health pyramid in the event of complications.

In terms of **clinical characteristics and** vaccination status, **the** majority of patients (95.8%) were correctly vaccinated according to the EPI. This result is higher than that of UNICEF Mali, which found that 45% of children had received all the basic vaccinations (41). Nutritional status showed that 5% of our patients were malnourished, of whom 2.9% had severe malnutrition and 2.1% moderate malnutrition. Our results are lower than those of the national survey, which found that 27% of children were chronically malnourished, 9% were acutely malnourished and 19% were underweight(42). This difference could be explained by the fact that the data were not collected in the nutrition departments.

The **paraclinical characteristics,** the CBC and CRP showed that a blood count had been carried out in 11.5% of our patients and 4.2% of cases had neutrophil hyperleukocytosis. CRP was performed in 6.9% of patients and was positive in 2.9%.

CSF ECB was performed in 6 patients (1.4%) and was positive in 4 patients (0.8%). The low rate of performance of these tests could be explained by their availability and the high cost of the tests, but also by the fact that they are not routinely performed in outpatients.

The RDT or thick drop was positive in 18 patients (3.7%). This result could be explained by the fact that the time of collection was not the peak malaria period.

In terms of antibiotic therapy, the prescription of antibiotic families shows that the most prescribed antibiotic families were beta-lactam antibiotics (80.9%), followed by aminoglycosides (22.2%), macrolides (13.3%) and nitroimidazoles

(7.2%). Our results are similar to those of Ouleymatou K (43) in 2022 in Bamako, with 36.9% of beta-lactams, followed by quinolones (33.4%) and macrolides (15.5%).At Sikasso Hospital, Kadidia Konate 2020 also found a high prescription rate for beta-lactams (58.5%), followed by nitroimidazoles (20.9%), aminoglycosides (16.2%) and quinolones (3.3%)(44). The predominance of beta-lactams may be due to their efficacy in treating frequent infections, their broad spectrum of action and good tolerance in children, and their lower cost. This widespread use of beta-lactam antibiotics could eventually lead to resistance and the abandonment of conventional beta-lactam antibiotics.

The association of antibiotics found that 14 molecules belonging to 9 families had been used. The majority of patients (72.4%) were on monotherapy and ceftriaxone was the most prescribed, accounting for 37.6% of prescriptions, followed by amoxicillin (28%) and 21.6%. gentamicin. Contrary to the results of O. Ikobo et al 2022 in Brazzaville, who found that gentamicin was prescribed predominantly in 92.7% of cases, followed by amoxicillin in 38.8%(45). A study carried out in early 2020 in Italy (46) showed that penicillin was prescribed predominantly in 52% of cases, followed by coamoxicillins in 33% and macrolides in 10%. The ceftriaxone +gentamicin combination was the most prescribed, accounting for 18.8% of cases. This combination was the most widely used in the study by Bamba A Sangaré(8).The majority of treatments (54.9%) lasted seven 7 days or less and in 16.4% of cases the duration was not mentioned. This result is similar to those found by Ciré et al (40) in Conakry with a duration of antibiotic therapy of less than or equal to seven 7 days in 73% of cases. This could be explained by the fact that the majority of patients were seen in consultation and did not require hospitalisation or had a severe infection requiring a long course of treatment. It is very important to be precise about the duration of treatment, as this allows the patient to observe the treatment and not stop it once the signs of infection have partially disappeared.With regard to the route of antibiotic administration, a preference for the oral route was observed. In fact, 63.4% of antibiotics prescribed were by this route, followed by 42.4% by the parenteral route and 2.9% by the local route. Our results are contrary to those of Diradourian et al (47) in 2022, who found that 77% of prescriptions were by the intravenous route. It is also contrary to that of M.N'fafing Sangaré (10) in 2022, who found that 65.8% of antibiotics were prescribed intravenously. Diallo et al(48) found in a study carried out in the paediatric ward of the Ratoma Community Medical Centre (CMC) that 87.4% of prescriptions were for oral antibiotics. The predominance of the oral route in our study could be explained by the fact that most of the patients were outpatients (92%) and that the oral route was easier to use and less expensive.

Signs of onset and hypothesis of diagnosis showed that fever was observed in 70.3% of cases, while the common cold (35.1%) and cough (37.8%) were the main signs of onset. These signs were related to the most common diagnoses, namely respiratory infections (30.3%), followed by tonsillitis (14.3%) and malaria (11.6%). The same observation was made by F. Messina et al (49) following a study carried out in Italy with 56% of respiratory tract infections and a predominance of 67.8% of acute otitis media.

In Mali in 2018, according to the 6th Demographic and Health Survey, 2% of children under the age of 5 showed symptoms of lower respiratory infections. Mali, like most countries in sub-Saharan Africa, records malaria as the leading cause of mortality and morbidity. In 2018, according to the health information system, 2,614,104 confirmed cases of malaria and 1,001 deaths were recorded. Malaria was the main reason for 39% of consultations(42). German data show that 70% of antibiotic prescriptions for children and adolescents under the age of 15 are for respiratory tract infections(46).

Assessment of the quality of prescriptions revealed that non-conformity with the RENAM and failure to indicate the dosage and duration of treatment were the causes of poor prescribing. Overall, the quality of prescription writing did not comply with the RENAM, and prescriptions were therefore judged to be of poor quality in 81% of cases. Bamba A Sangaré at CHU Gabriel Touré in 2020 found that in 68.3% of cases, antibiotic therapy was not adapted to national and/or international recommendations. Ouleymatou K (43) in 2022 found that 60.7% of prescriptions were of good quality.

CONCLUSION

At the end of the study, it was found that the main factors influencing the quality of antibiotic prescribing were prescribing, follow-up method, fathers' occupation and training in antibiotic therapy. Betalactam antibiotics were the most frequently prescribed. Similarly, it was found that antibiotic consumption was high in paediatrics, in both outpatient and inpatient settings. On the other hand, it was observed in the facilities visited that the majority of antibiotic prescriptions did not comply with the RENAM, and some prescriptions were made without confirmation of a clinical or paraclinical examination. Similarly, it was found that RENAM did not give either the dosage or the duration of antibiotic treatment. This could be because the RENAM gave neither the dosage nor the duration of antibiotic treatment for use in children. It would be desirable to revise this tool to make it complete in order to facilitate the implementation of actions to promote the proper use of antibiotics in paediatrics to ensure that children receive appropriate, high-quality care for their well-being.

REFERENCES

1. Brian J. Werth. MSD manuals for the general public. 2022 [cited 18 Jan 2024]. Antibiotics presentation - Infections. Available at: https://www.msdmanuals.com/fr/accueil/infections/antibiotiques/pr%C3%A9sent ation-des-antibiotiques

2. Masson E. EM-Consulte. 1994 [cited 18 Jan 2024]. Evolution of bacterial resistance to antibiotics. Available from: https://www.em-consulte.com/article/11783/evolution-de-la-resistance-bacterienne-aux- antibio

3. wikipedia. Antibiotic. In: Wikipedia [Internet]. 2023 [cited 17 Jan 2023]. Available from: https://fr.wikipedia.org/w/index.php?title=Antibiotique&oldid=200349724

4. Traore M. N. Evaluation de la prescription d'antibiotique chez les Patients en ambulatoires du CHU-CNOS de Bamako : à propos de 227 cas. [Internet] [Thèse medecine]. [Bamako]: USTTB; 2019 [cited 17 Jan 2023]. Available from: https://bibliosante.ml/bitstream/handle/pdf

5. ReAct [Internet]. [cited 23 Jan 2023]. National Action Plans on AMR. Available from: https://www.reactgroup.org/national-action-plans/

6. Da L, Somé D, Yehouenou C, Ouédraogo AS, Lienhardt C, Poda A. Current state of antibiotic resistance in sub-Saharan Africa. Médecine Mal Infect Form. 1 March 2023;2(1):3-12.

7. Mr KANTA Seydou. Antibiotic therapy in the paediatric department of the Gabriel Touré University Hospital in https://www.keneya.net/fmpos/theses/2008/pharma/pdf/

8. sangaré.B A. Analyse de la prescription des antibiotiques dans le département de Pediatrie du CHU Gabriel Toure Bamako, [Thèse de Médecine]. [Bamako]: USTTB; 2020 [cited 14 Jan 2023]. Available from: https://www.bibliosante.ml/bitstream/handle/

9. WHO. World Health Organization. 2020 [cited 17 Jan 2023]. Antibiotic Resistance. Available from: https://www.who.int/fr/news-room/fact-sheets/detail/antibiotic-resistance

10. SANGARE MN. ANALYSIS OF ANTIBIOTIC PRESCRIBING IN STRUCTURES HOSPITALIERES : CAS DU CHU HOPITAL DU MALI [Internet] [these de pharmacie]. [Bamako]: USTTB; 2022 [cited 14 Jan 2023]. Available from: https://www.bibliosante.ml/bitstream/handle/123456789/5393/22P11.pdf?sequen

ce=1&isAllowed=y

11. Armann J, Rüdiger M, Berner R, Mense L. Restrictive prescription of antibiotics in preterm infants with premature rupture of membranes. BMC Pediatr. 12 Jul 2022;22:408.

12. Hiddou A, Hamdani H, Elmouaych I, Zemmrani Y, Ahroui Y, Fouad A, et al. Evaluation of antibiotic prescribing in paediatric emergencies at the Mohammed VI University Hospital in Marrakech. J Pediatrics Childcare. March 1, 2018;31(1):34-9.

13. LAGNIKA Yazid Akin-Ola. ASSESSMENT OF ANTIBIOTIC PRESCRIBING AT THE DJEFFA HEALTH CENTRE. 2019;42.

14. WHO. World Health Organization. 2016 [cited 26 Oct 2023]. Global action plan to combat antimicrobial resistance. Available from: https://www.who.int/fr/publications-detail/9789241509763

15. O'Neill, Jim. Wellcome Collection. 2014 [cited 10 Nov 2023]. Antimicrobial resistance: tackling a crisis for the health and wealth of nations / the Review on Antimicrobial Resistance chaired by Jim O'Neill. Available from: https://wellcomecollection.org/works/rdpck35v

16. Yalcouye EY. Prescription des antibiotiques dans le Service d'Accueil des Urgences du CHU Gabriel Touré [Internet] [Thèse de medecine]. [Bamako]; 2020 [cited 14 Jan 2023]. Available from: https://www.bibliosante.ml/bitstream/handle/123456789/4099/20M268.pdf?seque nce=1&isAllowed=y

17. Ebongue CO, Tsiazok MD, Mefo'o JPN, Ngaba GP, Beyiha G, Adiogo D. Evolution of antibiotic resistance in enterobacteriaceae isolated at Douala General Hospital from 2005 to 2012. Pan Afr Med J [Internet]. 2015 [cited 17 Jan 2023];20. Available from: https://www.ncbi.nlm.nih.gov/pmc/articles/PMC4482524/

18. Larousse É. bactérie scientific Latin bacterium from Greek baktêrion little stick - LAROUSSE [Internet]. [cited 20 Sep 2023]. Available from: https://www.larousse.fr/encyclopedie/divers/bact%C3%A9rie/25038

19. Marouf manel -. Academia. 2014 [cited 9 Feb 2023]. Structure and physiology of bacteria : Anatomy - Structure |. Available from: https://www.academia.edu//Structure_et_physiologie_de_la_bacerie/Anatomie_St ructure

20. Futura. Futura. 2023 [cited 7 Feb 2023]. Bacteria. Available from: https://www.futura- sciences.com/health/definitions/medicine-bacteria-101/

21. VIDAL [Internet]. [cited 13 Jan 2023]. Antibiotic. Available from: https://www.vidal.fr/medicaments/utilisation/antibiotiques/antibiotiques-c-est-

quoi.html

22. Antibiotic. In: Wikipedia [Internet]. 2023 [cited 21 Sep 2023]. Available from: https://fr.wikipedia.org/w/index.php?title=Antibiotique&oldid=204404331

23. Antibiotics [Internet]. [cited 29 nov 2023]. List of Antibiotics. Available from: http://www.antibiotique.eu/liste-dantibiotiques.html

24. Antibiotics: modes of action, mechanisms of resistance - devsante.org [Internet]. [cited 7 Oct 2023]. Available from: https://devsante.org/articles/antibiotiques-modes-d-action-mecanismes-de-la-resistance/

25. Djaouida R. Antibiotics in veterinary medicine. :66.

26. Wikipedia. Prescription. In: Wikipedia [Internet]. 2020 [cited 1 Nov 2023]. Available from: https://fr.wikipedia.org/w/index.php?title=Prescription_(m%C3%A9decine)&oldid=176416528

27. Marion Berthon. Medical diagnostics [Internet]. 2020 [cited 2 Nov 2023]. Available from: https://www.deuxiemeavis.fr/blog/article/310-le-diagnostic-medical-les-etapes-pour-trouver-votre-maladie

28. Elsan [Internet]. 2023 [cited 2 Nov 2023]. ECBU. Available from: https://www.elsan.care/fr/pathologie-et- treatment/urinary-disease/ecbu-deroulement-interet

29. Hospitals M. Best Hospitals in India | Medicover Hospitals. [cited 2 nov 2023]. Cerebrospinal fluid (CSF) analysis | Medicover. Available from: https://www.medicoverhospitals.in/fr/diagnostics-pathology- tests/cerebrospinal-fluid-analysis

30. Tulkens PM. General Pharmacology of Antibiotics.

31. Antibiotic resistance. In: Wikipedia [Internet]. 2023 [cited 13 Oct 2023]. Available from: https://fr.wikipedia.org/w/index.php?title=R%C3%A9sistance_aux_antibiotiques&oldid=208461607

32. Gres E. Antibiotic prescribing practices according to the AWARE classification in children under five years of age at decentralised and hospital level in West Africa (2021-2022).

33. Veyssiere A. Antibiotic resistance in the bacteria most commonly encountered in community infections state of play in 2019.

34. FH. Mechanisms of resistance to anti-infective antibiotic agents [Internet]. 2022 [cited 13 Oct 2023]. Available from: http://aemip.fr/?page_id=3765

35. Antibiotic therapy: definition, duration, indications, principles [Internet]. 2022 [cited 12 Oct 2023]. Available from:

https://sante.journaldesfemmes.fr/fiches-medicaments/2803557-antibiotherapie-definition-indications/

36. Denes É, Hidri N. Synergy and antagonism in antibiotic therapy. Antibiotiques. May 2009;11(2):106-15.

37. FEDRAVET. Rules for the association of molecules [Internet]. Fedravet. [cited 12 Oct 2023]. Available from: https://fedravet.com/regles-d-association-des-molecules/

38. Sellam A, Chahwakilian P, Cohen R, Béchet S, Vie Le Sage F, Lévy C. [Impact of guidelines on ambulatory pediatric antibiotic prescriptions]. Arch Pediatr. 1 June 2015;22(6):595-601.

39. Adisa R, Orherhe OM, Fakeye TO. Evaluation of antibiotic prescriptions and use in under-five children in Ibadan, SouthWestern Nigeria. Afr Health Sci. Dec 2018;18(4):1189.

40. Ciré BM, Sidikiba S, Lamine DM, Bella S, Binta DF, Moustapha DM, et al. Prescription of antibiotics in the pediatric department of the Ignace Deen National Hospital in Conakry (Guinea) / Prescription des Antibiotiques dans le service de pédiatrique de l'Hôpital National Ignace Deen à Conakry (Guinée).

41. Fatou Diagne. UNICEF. [cited 23 Oct 2023]. Vaccines are free - yet some children don't get them. Available at: https://www.unicef.org/mali/recits/les-vaccins-sont-gratuits-pourtant- some-children-don't-receive-them.

42. INSTAT, CPS/SS-DS-PF and ICF. Mali Demographic and Health Survey 2018.6th edition. Bamako, Mali and Rockville, Maryland, USA; 2018.

43. KEITA O. PHARMACEUTICAL ANALYSIS OF ANTIBIOTIC PRESCRIBING IN PRIVATE PHARMACIES IN COMMUNE I OF THE DISTRICT OF BAMAKO. 2021;79.

44. Kadidia K. ANALYSIS OF ANTIBIOTIC PRESCRIPTION AT SIKASSO HOSPITAL [Thèse de medecine]. [Bamako]: USTTB; 2020.70p.

45. Ollandzobo Ikobo LC, Pea EA, Ngakengni NY, Ekouya Bowassa G, Mbika Cardorelle A. Prescription of antibiotics in neonates hospitalised in Brazzaville. J Pédiatrie Puériculture. 1 Feb 2022;35(1):29-35.

46. MSc JAB MPH, Malte Kohns Vasconcelos. Rational antibiotic treatment in paediatric practice [Internet]. paediatrics switzerland. 2023 [cited 18 Oct 2023]. Available from: https://www.paediatrieschweiz.ch/fr/traitement-antibiotique-rationnel-en-pratique-pediatrique/

47. Diradourian L, Walser S, Labrune P, Sandrine R, Lambert De Cursay C. Antibiotics in hospitalised children: evaluation of correct use and prescribing methods. Pharm Clin. 1 Dec 2022;57(4):e122-3.

48. Diallo ML, Barry IK, Camara E, Diallo SB, Bangoura K, Ondima LHM, et

al. Prescription des antibiotiqueschez les enfants de 0 a 14 ans au service depediatrie du Centre Medical Communal (CMC) de Ratoma. J Rech Sci L'Université Lomé. 2019;21(3):343-8.

49. Messina F, Clavenna A, Cartabia M, Piovani D, Bortolotti A, Fortino I, et al. Antibiotic prescription in the outpatient paediatric population attending emergency departments in Lombardy, Italy: a retrospective database review. BMJ Paediatr Open. 11 Dec 2019;3(1):e000546.

TABLE OF CONTENTS

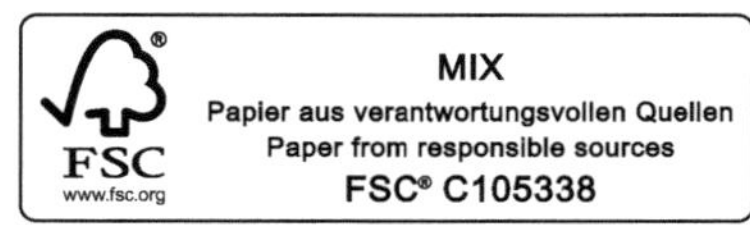